Pain Relief

THE DRUG-RREE WAY TO FEEL BETTER FAST

Maria Johnson

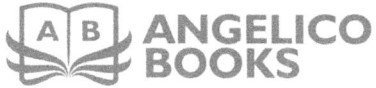

ANGELICO BOOKS

Table of Contents

Introduction
You Can Live a Pain-Free Life

You are reading this book for the same reasons that I am writing it: we are both victims of chronic pain. And like you, I have tried everything that modern medicine has to offer in order to manage it. I have taken pills and capsules of all colors and dosages. Like you, I have wished for my normal life—a life without pain—to come back.

Imagine waking up every day and feeling great; unlike now, when that uncomfortable sensation of pain serves as your alarm clock.

Imagine feeling free again: being able to use your body with the vigor and vitality of youth.

Imagine all the things you can do if only the pain would stop.

By the end of this book, I promise you: *you won't need to imagine.*

The road to a pain-free life is incredibly easy, practical, and realistic. And I am here to guide you on this road—think of me as your guide out of this murky jungle.

I discovered this method when I got tired of chugging down painkiller after painkiller. I went from doctor to doctor trying to find the best pill to ease my pain, accumulating dozens of bottles labeled with pharmacology words that I do not even understand.

Oh, the meds do work—but not in the way I want them. Sure, the pills eased the pains in my lower back, but I also felt groggy, sleepy, and drained of energy. In the end, I still wasn't able to function normally.

I knew that the pain was still there, just waiting to pounce once the meds wear off.

I drew the line when these pills affected my health. One of my allergies triggered, and the pill I took earlier worsened the effect: because painkillers slow down breathing, I was practically gasping for air and had to be taken to the hospital.

After that episode, I said goodbye to those multi-colored tablets. I threw away all my prescriptions, and tried to find a way to manage pain naturally.

I am now in my 60s, the age when you'd think my body would start developing all kinds of pain. But here I am, writing this book, not a single sensation of pain in my hand, and none throughout the rest of my body. I can jog, play with my grandkids, swing a perfect backhand, and not worry about feeling pain.

You can be the same.

You can spend your days without suffering long bouts of pain.

You can live your life to the fullest.

And the best part of it is you don't need to imagine—you can start your journey to a pain-free life by turning the pages.

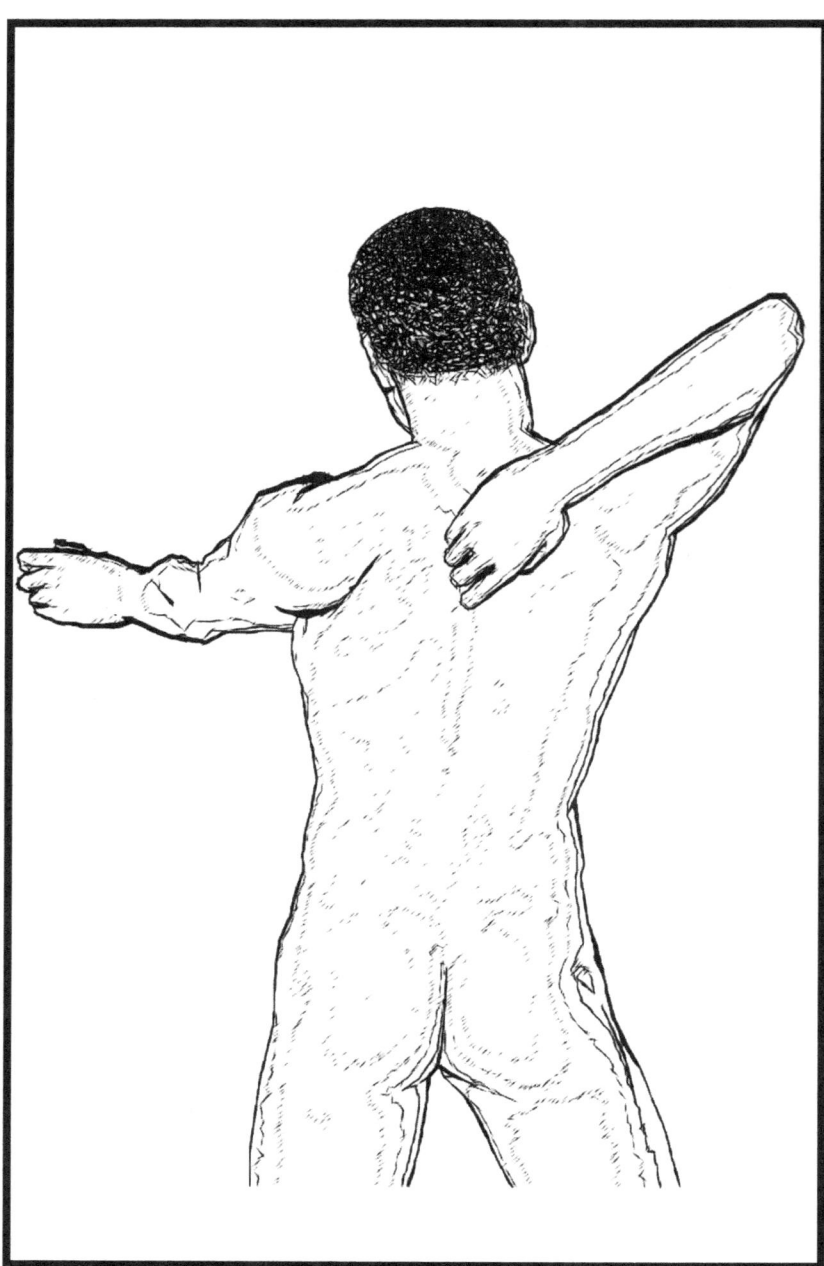

CHAPTER ONE

Understanding Pain

This book does not aim to replace your doctor's opinion. In fact, throughout this book, you will see several excerpts of research by renowned doctors and medical practitioners. After all, doctors do know best when it comes to how our body operates.

What this book aims to do is to change *you*—how you perceive, react to, and deal with pain. No matter how good your physician is, the biggest part of the equation in ending chronic pain is *you*.

The "Instant" Mindset

We all grew up in this fast-paced modern society where everything can be achieved in an instant. If you're hungry, just pop that mac & cheese into your microwave and you're all set. If you want to buy anything, just go online and you'll be able to with a few clicks of a mouse.

Whether we like it or not, we imbibed this "instant" mindset and we use it whenever we deal with pain. Because we are so used to having a fast solution to any inconvenience, we also expect an instant-off button to our migraine or backache.

So what do we do when we experience pain? We run to the nearest pharmacy and ransack the shelves with the most powerful painkillers that can take away the pain quickly. Headache? Take a double dose of Advil. Cramps? Take Ponstel.

This mindset is more damaging than helpful when it comes to pain. The meds may ease your pain now, but it does nothing to make you free from it in the long run. Long-term use of painkillers may cause even more horrible side-effects, from hormonal and chemical imbalances to an increase in tolerance and addiction, which can cause even more pain.

Pain as an Ally

A large reason why the painkiller culture we belong to is prevalent is due not understanding what pain really is. Most of us think that pain is something external to us; that it is something that we should want to live without.

The truth is that pain belongs to us. It is something internal, and it is something good.

The reason why the human race is still alive is because we have the capacity to feel pain. Without it, our species would have been extinct long ago. Without pain, you would not know that a knife is something that you should be careful with, or fire is something that you should not play with.

Pain is our body's way of warning us against physical harm. Those pangs of discomfort are your mind's way of telling you that something is dangerous to you and that you should avoid it.

Ever touched a really hot pot without any potholders? Remember how excruciating it felt? Well, thank your body for reacting the way it did: without pain, you would have continued on holding that hot pot, and you would incur major burns.

Pain is there to tell you: *something's not right and you should fix it.*

Extinguish the Fire, Not the Smoke

Here's something that sounds absurd, but is 100% true: Painkillers are not the answer to pain. Yes, you read that right. All these pills do not provide a solution to the cause of the pain; they just provide a temporary screen that filters the sensation.

As you have learned from this chapter, pain is not the problem; it is your body's way of saying that there's a deeper issue.

Pain is not the fire; it is the smoke that warns you of the existence of fire. In a burning room, your main concern should not be how to get rid of all the suffocating smoke; it's how to extinguish the fire that produces the smoke in the first place.

It's the same in your body. *The best way to get rid of pain completely is to find the core problem and fix it.*

4

Chapter Two

Five Simple Steps to Feeling Better

But what if the problem isn't that easy to fix?

Chronic pain, such as what I and several of the clients I have life-coached experienced, is due to a problem that is recurrent and has no permanent solution. Arthritis, migraine, and menstrual cramps are just some of the illnesses that my clients had to deal with. Like you, they have drowned themselves in medication whenever they experience debilitating pain.

That is, until I have shared with them what I did with my own problem with pain—they followed my five simple steps towards feeling better and healthier.

When I say simple, I do really mean *simple*. These are ways that have been proven effective for centuries, since the earliest days of civilization, even before modern medicine produced the first painkiller. They are too familiar, such that they are disregarded. Yet they are invaluable. And here they are:

The Five Simple Steps to being Pain-Free

- Drinking lots of water

- Getting plenty of sleep

- Exercising regularly

- Strengthening the mind to strengthen the body

- Having the right hormonal and nutritional support

I can sense your apprehension right now. Do you find these too simple? Too trivial? Too cliché?

When I uncovered these steps, I was apprehensive too. I spent a great deal of time, effort, and energy trying to find an alternative to painkillers, and all my research ends up at these really simple things—things that I have known all my life, and are staring me right at the face.

At first, I just couldn't accept it. During the first months of me doing these steps, I was still furiously researching, trying to see if I missed something. And then I noticed... I wasn't feeling pain anymore. Not when I wake up, not when I do my morning exercise, not when I play tennis. And no, it's not similar to the temporary relief that painkillers provide. I could feel that I was free from pain. *It just worked.*

The road to ending your pain and feeling good again is supposed to be as simple as that. It doesn't need to be complex. It doesn't need to be scientifically intimidating. It doesn't need to be expensive. It doesn't need to be hard to find nor hard to do. *It just needs to work no matter how simple it is.*

In the next few pages, I will share with you not only the science of these simple steps, but I will also provide help on how to do these steps in a correct manner.

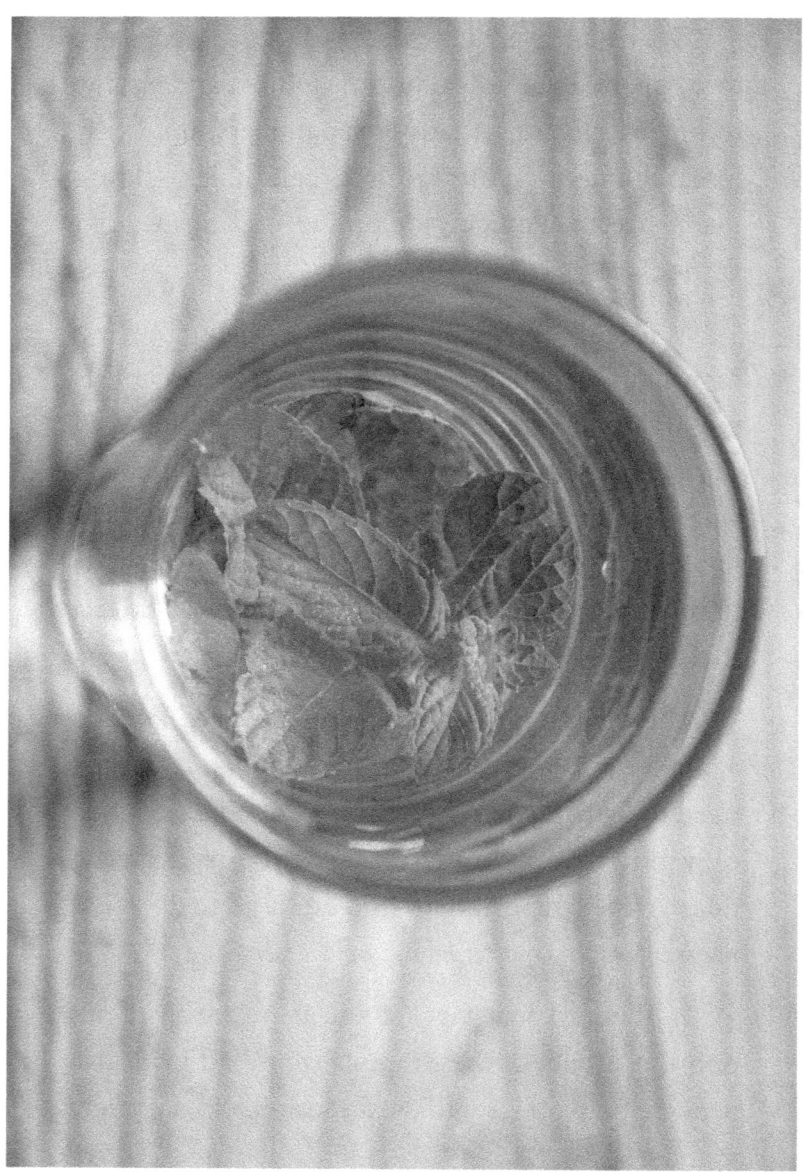

Chapter Three

Water as a Miracle Cure

There's a reason why water was dubbed as the elixir of life. Its mystery, as romanticized by many great poets and adventurers, is beyond myth. Water is a source of life. It is a natural cure for any pain.

Your body needs water to perform its fundamental functions and to maintain its natural balance. Without water, your body breaks down. You become dehydrated and you will feel pain in all parts of your body.

Here is a list of common bodily pains you might be suffering from:

- Heartburn

- Lower back pain

- Migraine

- Rheumatoid arthritis

- Dyspepsia

- Fibromyalgia

- Colitis

- Angina

These illnesses have one thing in common: one of its causes is the *insufficiency of water in our body.*

In fact, a person would probably have not suffered these illnesses were they drinking plenty of water every day. Surprised that it's as simple as that?

The Magic of Water

Water, the most abundant substance on earth, is also the most abundant substance in our body. Water is a life-giving substance and very essential to all the metabolic processes in our body.

Here are some of the things that water does for our body:

- Delivers nutrients to cells, and transports wastes away from cells. It also transports essential substances such as enzymes, hormones, blood cells, and blood platelets.

- Makes our body free from waste through a complicated process of chemical reaction. The end result: urine.

- Serves as the oil of our body: Water is a vital component in the natural lubricating fluids for joints, digestive tracts, and other internal organs.

- Regulates body temperature by absorbing heat and releasing it through perspiration.

- Maintains cellular shape and cell membrane. Healthy cells = healthy body.

- In addition, water cushions organs and maintains body structures.

Our body needs to maintain enough amount of water to function properly. Remember that we lose water through various means—and we're not only talking about perspiration here, but also when the body uses water internally for its processes. When the amount of water loss is excessive, our body automatically signals its need for water through different kinds of pain. This mechanism enables our body to maintain water balance until replenishment arrives.

The importance of water in our body and how it works is like perfectly designed machinery. Our body needs water to function properly. If you are almost always feeling pain, your body might be screaming to be hydrated.

There is No Substitute for Water

In our modern society, it's so easy to forego drinking water as we have so many alternative and tastier thirst-quenchers. We have soda, energy drinks, tea... and you're probably aware of the marketing campaign that sports drinks have: they're better than water.

While that may be true to some degree when it comes to quenching thirst quickly, it isn't true when it comes to our body. Nothing can be better for our body than water.

And while that sports drink might taste better than plain old water, it also causes more stress to your bodily functions. Just think of how much flavoring, sugar, food coloring, and other chemicals there are to make that sports drink look and taste appealing. The sports drink might have some more electrolytes, but the other stuff that comes with it are unnecessary for your body.

Water is the purest way to hydrate your body. It doesn't add stress to your digestive system, and it doesn't make your metabolic functions go into overdrive.

How Water can Ease Pain and Illnesses

Are you still not a fan of this tasteless and clear liquid called water? Here are some of the ways that water eases pain and illnesses:

1. **Water boosts your endurance.** Your body spends a lot of glycogen—a form of energy your muscles use during exercise. When you drink a lot of water, your body spends less glycogen because it will use the fluid you

have taken in. More glycogen in your body means more energy to be used for all kinds of activities.

2. **Water can beat the common colds.** According to Dr. Kenneth Lem, a clinical pharmacy lecturer at the University of California in San Francisco, water is the best expectorant if you have colds. That's because one of the major cause of colds and cough is the lack of water that dries out the mucus-producing tissues that coats your throat.

3. **Water can cure stomachaches caused by medicines or food.** An Advil or any aspirin brand may be really effective for head-splitting headaches, but you sometimes have the added side-effect of stomach pains. Drinking enough water will dilute and dissolve the medicine so it won't be strong enough for your stomach to handle. The same is true if you have hyper-acidity or food poisoning—water helps your stomach sort out the problem with less pain.

4. **Hydrate, and fly without experiencing jet-lag.** You might think that it's just a time-zone

thing. Actually, dehydration occurs during air flights because the dry air inside the plane caused by the low level of oxygen can suck water out of your system. This results to fatigue during and after your flight. An extra glass of water before your flight and another one after your flight can help you prevent the feeling of jetlag during air travel.

5. **Water prevents bowel problems.** If you don't drink water you will likely get constipated. To treat constipation, you need to drink lots of water in order to flush the solid wastes that have gotten stuck in your bowels. Further, if you experience loose bowel movement or diarrhea, the best advice any doctor can give you is to drink plenty of water. As much as possible, you will need to drink as much water as you can in order to replenish the lost fluids caused by LBM or diarrhea.

6. **Water prevents kidney and urinary problems.** It is a known fact that kidney stones and major urinary problems can be prevented and cured with water. Research headed by Dr. Gary Curhan, MD, a nephrologist and

epidemiologist from Boston's Brigham and Women's Hospital, suggested that 8 to 10 glasses of water a day can significantly decrease the chances of having kidney stones.

7. **Water freshens up your tired mind.** Dehydration can have an adverse effect in your ability to think and make decisions properly. This is because while dehydrated, all your body's energy is being spent in regulating your body. So if you are writing your report and you experience a mental block, don't drink coffee—it will only make you more dehydrated. Drink water instead.

8. **Water helps regulate your body temperature.** Pain is often caused by inflammation—a topic we will discuss later on. But for now, the only thing you need to know is that one of the reasons why inflammation hurts is because of the increased temperature around the inflamed area. One way to bring down this temperature—and in effect, lessen the pain—is to drink plenty of water. Hydrate, and your body will do the rest.

9. **Water helps you regulate your weight.** Most of the common body pains that adults experience are due to the stress that our weight adds to our joints or muscles. But did you know that thirst could often be misinterpreted as hunger? That's according to research by Nautilus Sports and Medical Industries' former director of research, Dr. Ellington Darden, PhD. He also added that drinking eight pints of ice water per day could actually help you drop a pound every month.

Making Sure You are Hydrated

We have all heard that good old doctor's advice about drinking 8 to 10 glasses of water a day. While that is true, being hydrated is not only an issue of the *amount* of water you drink; it is also an issue of frequency: how often a person drinks water.

If you neglect drinking water for four hours straight (which is half a working day), then drink three glasses at one go, you still wouldn't be properly hydrated. There is only so much water the body can process in a span of time—drink too much, and most of it goes to waste.

So how can you make sure that you are hydrated? Here are three simple things you can do:

1. **Take an hourly water break.** That's what your water cooler tank in the office is for anyway. Not only are you hydrating, but you are also doing your mind a favor: a break of a few minutes from number crunching or looking at the monitor makes you stay sharp. But even when you're at home and relaxing on your couch, you still should follow these hourly hydration breaks.

2. **When doing physical activities, drink 2–3 times the normal amount of water.** Physical activities drain water from your body not only to regulate heat (which is why you perspire), but also to use in energy production. Even if the only exercise you do is a simple round-the-block jog, you need to replace the water that's already been used *plus interest*. You need that extra water to fight the lactic acid produced

by your sore muscles, which is what makes your body ache badly after a hard workout.

3. **Do NOT wait for thirst.** Thirst, like pain, is the body's way of telling you that you are dehydrated; which means you are already *lacking* water when you feel thirsty. Under no circumstances should you wait for that dry feeling in your throat before you drink water.

Trust me, if you religiously drink water, your pain will be decreased significantly. It is a pretty simple task, which I am sure you can do without fail.

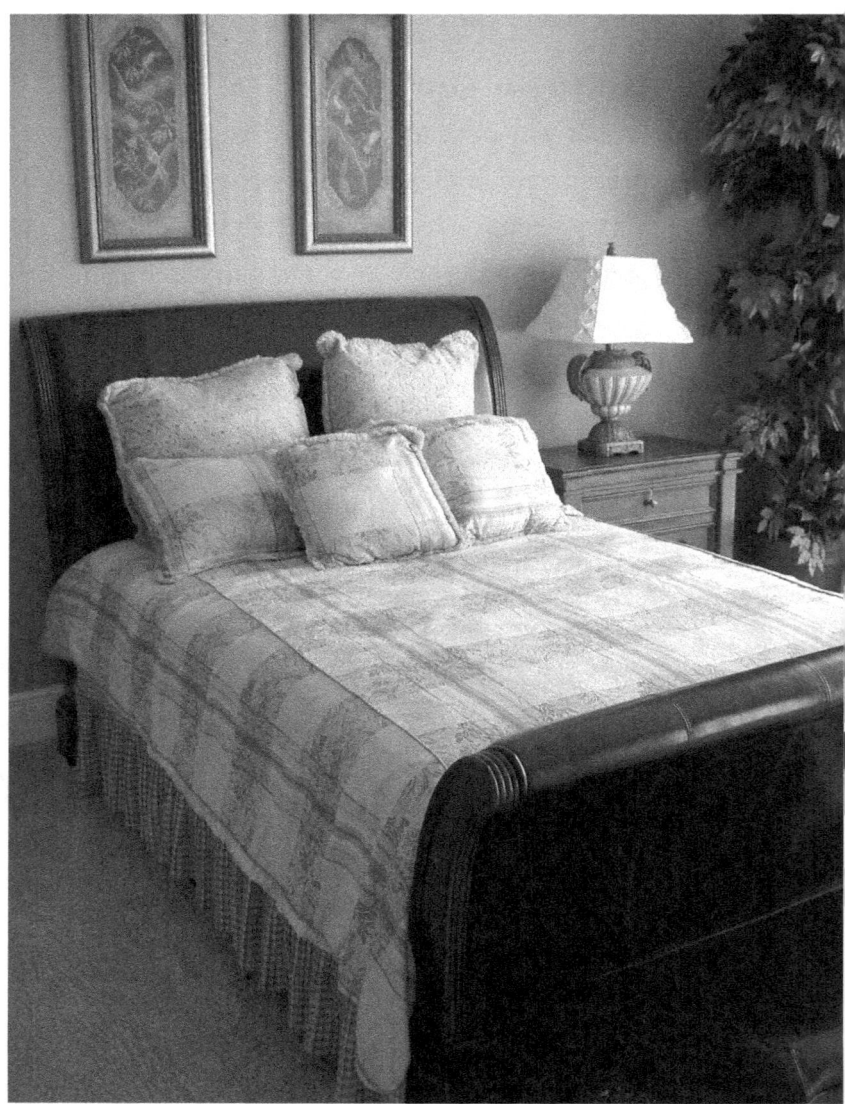

Chapter Four

Sleep as a Natural Way of Healing

In the modern world where long work hours, deadlines, and stress are the norm, people tend to overlook the importance of sleep. Most successful individuals have cut sleep in their daily routine in order to maximize the time they spend on their careers. Unfortunately, the toll of the lack of sleep on their health is something they will soon regret.

Take one of my clients as an example. Max, who works at a marketing agency, came to me for help in feeling physically better. He is incredibly good at what he does, thus, he gets more clients and assignments than most people in his company. Max is happy with this, of course, but he felt as if the 24 hours that we have in a day is not enough—he wants to be able to do more, and thus spends countless hours at work. He sleeps for just two to three hours a day, as he thinks that sleep is the most inefficient use of his time.

And yet, this routine had a debilitating effect on him. Every day he experienced the worst kind of muscle and joint pain. His answer to this, of course, is to add pain killers in his daily diet. The pain goes away momentarily, but he noticed that it seems like it gets stronger and stronger as each day goes by. Not only that, but it seems he always gets some minor illness: a cold this week, coughs the other, fever the next. He had enough when he needed to back down on handling a big event because he just fell so physically unwell.

Max's doctor, of course, said that he needed take some rest. Not accepting this as the right solution to his woes, he came to me.

Can you guess what I said to Max?

Sleep as an Essential Part of Living

Think about your car. It might be able to run several miles straight, but it surely needs to rest after that long haul. Otherwise, you will be stressing out the engine severely, and the car will give up on you.

The human body is far more complex than a car sporting a V8, and yet the need for rest is quite similar. With not enough sleep, your body reacts negatively to the abuse, resulting in the following:

- muscle aches
- headaches
- increased blood pressure
- memory lapses
- additional stress hormone production

Additionally, if you lack sleep all the time, you are more prone to having serious illnesses such as diabetes, obesity, and depression.

The pain you are experiencing due to the lack of sleep is your body telling you to stop punishing it, and that it needs rest. So why not let it rest?

How Sleep Helps in Easing Pain and Illnesses

Let's go back to Max's story. I told Max that he should try to listen to his doctor's advice and get enough sleep every day, even just for a straight week. And while he protested at first, citing these reasons convinced him to try it:

1. **Sleep improves your immune system.** Several experiments have been conducted by scientists that have shown a significant decrease in white blood cell production (the cells that protect you from diseases) when you are sleep deprived. Conversely, white blood cell production is shown to be healthy when a person gets a good amount of sleep.

2. **Restorative processes work faster during sleep.** Several studies have shown that wound healing is affected by sleep—get enough shut-eye, and your body will heal your wounds faster. The same is true for any kind of injury or pain: broken bones, sore muscles, or internal injuries.

3. **Sleep preserves your energy.** While seemingly obvious, the fact that sleep conserves and preserves your energy is perhaps the biggest help that it will give you to combat pain. Ever wonder why you get incredibly hungry and thirsty when you are sleep deprived, and yet still feel weak after eating a lot? It's because your body can only store so much energy at one time. Sleep allows you to preserve enough energy to be used throughout the day. Plus, not only do you give time for restorative processes to work when you sleep, your body also gains enough energy so those processes continue to work at maximum efficiency during your waking hours.

After a week, Max gave me a call, telling me he's never felt better. All his aches are gone, and he felt stronger than before, both in body and mind.

The Secrets to Sleeping Well in the Presence of the Pain

Some of you who are reading this might be asking: "How can I sleep well if I'm in pain?" Or: "My arthritis just wakes me up in the dead of the night; how can you tell me that sleep is the answer if my pain isn't allowing me to sleep?"

I've been there. I have woken up in the middle of the night, sweating profusely because of the pain in my back. The fact that lying down applies pressure on my back doesn't help the case.

Through my research, I found several methods that are extremely effective at letting me sleep without the worry that my pain will somehow wake me up (or prevent me from sleeping at all). And while some of these may seem tedious to do, the payoff is worth the effort. Not only will you get enough sleep, but because you get well-rested, the pain you are experiencing will decrease over time.

Secret 1: Create a Sleep Ritual

You might think that sleeping is as simple as lying down on the bed and closing your eyes. The truth is more complex: your body needs to be prepared in order for you to get a really good sleep. You need to tell your body that it should wind down all its processes and relax.

Stanford University Center for Sleep Sciences and Medicine fellow Brandon Peters, M.D. defines sleep as a physiological process highly dependent on behavior. He declares sleep as, *"a chance for rest that conserves energy and an opportunity to process memories and improve learning—but it is also a behavior."*

A good sleeping ritual is a key to having <u>restorative rest</u> that can heal whatever pain you are experiencing.

Dr. Peters adds:

In a very real sense our bodies can learn to sleep well, and we can also learn to sleep poorly. Our body follows a natural circadian rhythm, and by keeping a consistent sleep schedule, we can reinforce this. As part of better sleep guidelines, we can make other choices—including establishing a bedtime routine— that likewise improve our sleep patterns.

The essential part of having a sleeping ritual is how it serves to wind down both your body and mind. Here are some steps in creating your perfect sleep ritual:

1. **Your aim should be to make your senses and functions rest in a gradual manner. Start with your sense of taste and smell, and your**

digestive functions. You should make it a point to have your last full meal for the day two hours before your intended sleep time. Avoid drinking coffee or alcohol, and smoking. An hour before you sleep, you can drink something that will relax your taste, smell, and digestive functions. For most people, this means warm milk or hot tea.

2. **Next, you can make your muscles and your sense of touch relax by cleaning up.** Take a fifteen-minute soak in the bathtub, or a long hot shower. The key here is to take your time— taking a quick shower stimulates your senses and wakes you up, but a long soak will make you relax.

3. **Go to your room and either read a book or listen to soft music.** Either means either: you must choose; you cannot do both at the same time. Your aim is to make either your sense of sight or your sense of hearing rest. (This is why you should never watch television before you sleep—it stimulates both sight and hearing.) Go for what relaxes you better. If you go for reading a book, make sure that your room

is pretty quiet. And if you want to listen to music, try to dim the lights to give your eyes less stimuli. <u>Don't overdo this.</u> The book you are reading might be so engrossing, but you should put it down after about fifteen minutes. The same goes with your radio or mp3 player: gradually lower the volume, eventually switching it off after about fifteen minutes. You should not be falling asleep at this point; you should just be incredibly relaxed. If you are already at the brink of sleep when you close that book, you've probably overdone it.

4. **Turn off the lights, close your eyes, and let your mind wander off.** This is the crucial step that most people skip. By turning off the lights and closing your eyes, you are letting the last of your senses rest, but your mind is probably still active. You already took a lot of burden off your mind by making your senses relax one by one, but you won't be helping it fully rest by thinking about what your plans are for tomorrow. Instead, don't think about anything specific—just let your mind wander off. *Don't think about letting your mind wander off;* just let it be.

5. **If you can't relax due to pain, try meditation.**
   If you find that none of the steps above are
   helping you relax because of pain, try medi-
   tating before doing the above steps. A large
   part of pain is due to your mind not taking
   enough control over your body. Later in this
   book, you will learn about how the mind can
   be a great ally in pain management.

Secret 2: Sleeping and Waking Up at the Right Time

Your body has a natural clock called the *circadian
clock*. This is how your body knows when to do certain
actions and how to allot energy throughout the different parts of the day.

If you wake up, say, at around 7AM, your body
would work to give you the highest alertness possible
at around 10AM, the fastest reaction time at around
3PM, and the greatest muscle strength at around 5PM.

This is also true for sleeping. Even without doing
your sleeping ritual, your body starts to wind down on
its own at around 14 hours after you have woken up.

Syncing your sleep with your internal clock is part
of a good sleep routine. In fact, going to bed early is

not really the way for you to have a real good sleep; instead, it's going to bed *at the right time*.

Waking up at the right time is also crucial. Ever slept for 10 hours and felt horrible after waking up? This is because you have woken up in the middle of your sleep cycle. You see, our body has several sleep cycles during the night, characterized by non-rapid eye movement and rapid eye movement (REM) stages. A well-rested sleep consists of around 5 tc 6 cycles. Ideally, you should wake up sometime after you experience the last REM stage and before you experience another REM stage. Setting your alarm clock at a later or an earlier time makes you wake up not only grumpy, but probably in pain too.

But how would you know *when* to wake up? Thankfully, technology has given us the tools to help in managing our sleep. If you have an iPhone or an Android phone, there are several apps in the marketplace that adjusts your alarm depending on the time you sleep, so you can wake up in the right time.

You can also visit www.sleepyti.me. This website has a sleep cycle calculator: input the time when you need to wake up and it will tell you what time you need to sleep.

If you like things done manually, computing for your optimum waking or sleeping time is easy. Each sleep cycle lasts about around 90 minutes or so. If you want to know what time it is best to wake up, just mark every 90 minutes after your intended time of sleep. If you need to wake up at a specific time, count 90 minutes backward to get what time you need to sleep.

Knowing your circadian rhythm and having your sleep cycle schedule is really handy when experiencing chronic pain. Because you have a schedule, you will know when to prepare your body to relax, and when to do simple routines to lessen the pain before getting ready to sleep.

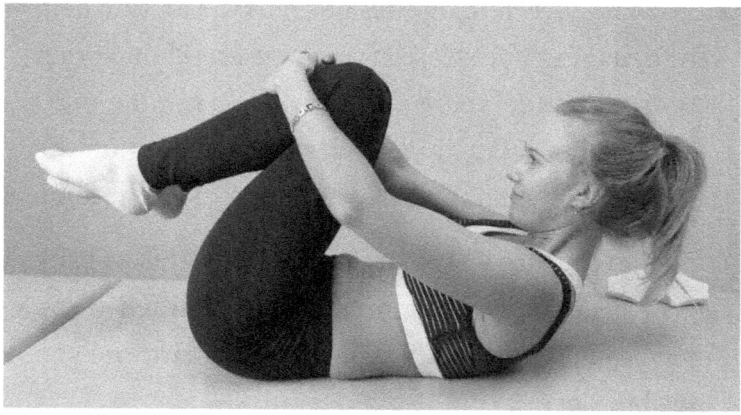

Chapter Five

Exercise as a Crucial Part of Rehabilitation

Exercise is the easiest way to prevent and treat pains. More often than not, the pains that you feel in specific parts of your body are caused by tissues and muscles that have become tensed, strained, or even shortened.

If your body lacks the exercise it requires to stay healthy and fit, you'll likely experience pains in parts of your body. A simple walk around the neighborhood will be a cause of sore muscles for a person who does not exercise.

The typical pains that you experience normally occur in your back area, your wrists, your joints, your knees, your neck and shoulders, your head, and other limbs. If you are experiencing these kinds of pain, the following exercise procedures will help to gradually relieve you of pain.

Back Pain Exercises

Your chronic back pain is best prevented and treated with exercise. Back exercises can strengthen the muscles that support your spine. This prevents, lessens, and—in most cases—eliminates lower back pain.

The major root of your lower back pain is, most often, weak <u>core muscles</u>. These are the muscles located at your back, hips, buttocks and abdomen. These core muscles are responsible for protecting your spine against gravity.

On top of that, your core muscles ensure correct posture and stabilize your spine to keep it firm and in its normal alignment during any of your movements—exercising, running, lifting, and walking, among others. Improving your core muscles also reduces your risk of injury in your back muscles and ligaments, spinal joints and discs during those activities.

You can relieve that lower back pain caused by shortened muscles by doing some stretching.

(Do you have any existing back injury or condition? Stop right here and call your physiotherapist; ask if a little exercise is okay with your injury or condition.)

Types of Back Pain Exercises

There are three major types of back pain exercises that you can do. Those would be stretching, strengthening and balancing, and stability exercises.

Stretching exercises can aid in lengthening your tight muscles. Examples of this are pelvic tilts, knee-to-chest stretches, and cobras.

Strengthening exercises are primarily targeted for your abdominals. Some examples are bridges, planks, and wall squats.

Balancing and stability exercises can aid in strengthening your deep core muscles which you primarily use for balancing. An example of this kind of exercise is the opposite arm and leg raise.

I have a simple routine here that can help you prevent back pains. Try my 15 minute every day back workouts below:

KNEE-TO-CHEST STRETCH

- Lie on your back: knees bent and feet flat on the floor.

- Use both hands to pull up one knee and press it towards your chest.

- Hold it up for 15 to 30 seconds then return to the starting point.

- Repeat with your opposite leg.

- Repeat both stretches at least twice or thrice—most recommended once in the morning and once in the evening.

LOWER BACK ROTATIONAL STRETCH

- Lie on your back: knees bent and feet flat on the floor.

- Keep your shoulders firmly on the floor and roll your bent knees to the right side.

- Hold it up for 10 seconds then return to the starting point.

- Repeat on the left side.

- Repeat both stretches at least twice or thrice—most recommended once in the morning and once in the evening.

LOWER BACK FLEXIBILITY WORKOUT

- **Lie on your back: knees bent and feet fl**at on the floor.

- Arch your back so that you can feel like your pubic bone is pointing towards your feet.

- Hold it up for 5 seconds then relax. Flatten your back, pulling your bellybutton towards the floor—so that you can feel like your pubic bone is pointing towards your head.

- Hold it up for 5 seconds then relax. Repeat. Start this with five repetitions every day and gradually work up to 30 repetitions.

BRIDGE WORKOUT

- Lie on your back: knees bent and feet flat on the floor.

- Keep your shoulders and your head relaxed on the floor and tighten your gluteal and abdominal muscles. Form a straight line from your knees to your shoulders by raising your hips.

- Hold that position long enough to complete three deep breaths. Return to your starting position. Start this with five repetitions every day and gradually work up to 30 repetitions.

CAT STRETCH

- Position yourself with your hands and knees on the floor.

- Let your back as well as your abdomen sag toward the floor slowly.

- Slowly arch your back by pulling your abdomen upwards toward the ceiling.

- Return to your starting position. Repeat this three to five times, twice a day.

SEATED LOWER BACK ROTATIONAL STRETCH

- Sit on an armless stool or chair. Cross your right leg over your left leg. Brace your elbow against the outside of your right knee. Twist and stretch to the side.

- Hold that for 10 seconds and then repeat on the opposite side.

- Repeat the stretch three to five times on both sides, twice a day.

SHOULDER BLADE SQUEEZE

- Sit on an armless stool or chair.

- Keep your chin tucked in as well as your chest high and then pull your shoulder blades together.

- Hold it up for five seconds and then relax. Repeat that three to five times and twice a day.

- Make sure to do that routine regularly to avoid the onset of any back related pain. It would just take you 15 minutes to do all the exercise.

Knee Pain Exercises

The best medicine for your knee pains is exercise. Dr. Willibald Nagler, M.D., head of the rehabilitation medicine at the New York Presbyterian Hospital-Cornell Campus, advises that strengthening the muscles around the joint protects you from injury by decreasing stress on the knee.

What you must keep in mind when doing exercises for knee pain is using a good form and technique.

This is the commandment that you need to learn by heart about knee pain exercises: *Don't bend your legs to the point where your knees stick out past your toes.* Not only that, apply this commandment when stretching and doing other aerobic exercises.

To alleviate the pain in your knees, here are some of my recommended exercises:

PARTIAL SQUATS

- Stand around 12 inches away from the front of a chair with your feet approximately hip width apart and your toes frontward.

- Bend your hips and gradually lower yourself halfway down to the chair. Make sure to maintain your abs tight and ensure your knees stay behind your toes.

STEP-UPS

- You would need an aerobic step bench or just a staircase to do this. Step up onto the step with your right foot.

- Then tap your left foot on the top of the step and then lower. As you step up, your knee should be directly over your ankle.

- Repeat that step with your left foot.

SIDE-LYING LEG LIFTS

- You would have to wear ankle weights above your knee to do this. Lie on your left side and support your head with your left arm; make sure to keep your legs straight and together.

- Slowly raise your right leg to about the height of your shoulder then lower gradually. Make sure your right foot is flexed and your body is straight while doing this.

- Repeat that step with your left leg.

INNER-THIGH LEG LIFTS

- You would need to wear ankle weights above your knee to do this. Lie on your left side; make sure it is slightly back your butt.

- Now, bend your right leg and position it at the back your left leg with your right foot flat on the floor and your left leg straight. Support your head using your left arm.

- Gradually lift your left leg for about 3 to 5 inches and then lower it slowly. Now repeat the steps with your right leg.

CALF RAISES

- Grab a chair or stand next to the wall, this is necessary for your balance, and stand with your feet around hip width apart, your toes should be straight ahead.

- Now, slowly lift your heels off the floor while rising up onto your toes.

- Hold it for a couple of seconds then lower slowly.

STRAIGHT-LEG RAISES

- You need to sit with your back against the wall. Lift your leg straight. Your right leg should be bent with your foot firmly flat on the floor.

- Slowly lift your left leg straight up for about 12 inches off the floor.

- Hold it up and the lower it slowly.

- Repeat the same step with your right leg.

SHORT-ARC KNEE EXTENSIONS

- Position yourself in the same starting position with the straight-leg raises.

- Put a ball the size of a regular basketball under your left knee so that your leg will be bent. Straighten your leg slowly.

- Hold it and then lower again slowly.

- Repeat the same step with your right leg.

HAMSTRING STRETCH

- Lie on the floor with your back and left leg flat on the floor.

- Now, loop a towel or rope around your right foot and pull your leg as far as comfortable towards your chest at the same time keeping a slight bend at your knee.

- Make sure to keep your back pressed to the floor throughout the whole stretch.

- Hold that position for 10 to 30 seconds and then release.

- You need to repeat that step three or four times with each leg. I advise you to do this stretch five or six times a week.

If you feel really enthusiastic about these very easy exercises to prevent and alleviate knee pains, I suggest you do those steps as relaxed and as comfortable as possible. Do not overdo your knee workout.

If you feel like you are overdoing your workout, go back again to your main goal which is to prevent and eliminate pain. As soon as you feel tense, discomfort, or even a little pain while doing the exercise, *stop and breathe before going back to the top.*

Now, go ahead and try them!

Wrist Pain Exercises

Your wrist is the most likely and accidentally injured part of your body. If you sit the whole 8 hours of your day job beating the keyboard like a professional percussionist, then you'll most likely develop wrist pains.

One of the most frequent wrist pains that you can develop would be the carpal tunnel syndrome. This kind of injury is common to people who use the computer for hours as well as those who make use too much of their hands at work.

There are some basic exercises that I can teach you to prevent and alleviate wrist pains caused by any conditions. So if you are ready now, prepare yourself in your most comfortable workout position and follow me.

WRIST FLEXION AND EXTENSION

- Start by supporting your forearm with a table or bench. Your wrist and fingers should be over the edge.

- Bend your wrist back and forth until you can sense a mild to moderate pain-free stretch.

- Repeat 10 times.

FOREARM ROTATION

- Start with your elbow on your side bent to a 90 degree angle.

- Rotate your palm upwards and downwards pain-free as much as possible.

- Repeat 10 times.

WRIST SIDE BENDS

- Start with your forearm supported by a bench or table with your wrist and fingers over the edge.

- Bend your wrist from sideward until you can feel a mild to moderate pain-free stretch.

- Repeat 10 times.

WRIST EXTENSOR STRETCH

- Holding your elbow straight, bend your wrist down using your other hand until you can feel a mild to moderate pain-free stretch.

- Hold for 15 seconds and then repeat 4 times.

WRIST FLEXOR STRETCH

- Holding your elbow straight, take your wrist toward the back using your other hand until you can feel a mild to moderate pain-free stretch.

- Hold for 15 seconds and then repeat 4 times.

Do you feel better now that you've performed these wrist exercises? Always make sure to do the workout as relaxed as possible to avoid straining your wrist and fingers.

Neck and Shoulder Pain Exercises

Have you been suffering from neck and shoulder tension? I know how painful and energy draining that is.

If you suffer from tension in that area, it's likely that you are putting too much strain on other parts of your body in order to get rid of the pain.

Before I lay down the easy ways to relieve neck and pain discomforts, I advise you to incorporate what I will be sharing with you to your daily routine. You'll thank me later on as soon as you start to feel the benefits of these exercises after a few days.

NECK ROLL

- You need to sit with your back straight on a chair; or you can stand upright with your feet a little bit apart and your knees a little bit bent. Relax your shoulders in a manner that you can feel that they are sinking down onto the ground. Relax your body while keeping your tummy in and your back straight.

- Stretch your neck upward cautiously and gradually while you sink your chin until it touches your chest, allowing your jaw to relax and hang freely.

- Relax your shoulders while you try to hold them a little backward.

- Now turn your head cautiously and slowly toward the right, keeping your chin down, until your nose is parallel with the center of your right shoulder.

- While you are holding this position, look over your shoulder as far as you can and try to stretch your neck even more. Hold that position while you count to five.

- While maintaining your neck stretched as much as possible - turn your head back to the middle position where you started off.

- Now turn your head in a similar way over to the left in an even, careful and slow movement. As soon as your nose is parallel with the center of your left shoulder, look over your shoulder as far as you can as you stretch your neck even more. Hold this position while you count to five.

- While you maintain your neck stretched – turn your head and chin back to the middle position.

- Start with two repetitions, gradually increasing per day, until you reach five repetitions.

NECK STRETCH

- Position yourself in a sitting position with your straight back on a chair, or you can stand upright with your feet a bit apart and your knees a bit bent. Make sure to relax your shoulders and arms.

- You can begin by stretching your neck upward until you can feel that you can no longer stretch any further. While doing that, make sure to relax your face and specifically your jaw. Now, close your eyes and imagine that your shoulders are slowly sinking down into the ground, and that there's an imaginary cord attached to the ceiling that is pulling your head up so that your neck is being stretched further. Now try to set that image into reality:

allow your shoulders to become heavy and drop while your neck is stretching upward as much as you can.

- This time turn your head carefully and gradually toward the right until you can feel it stretch. Hold the position for a few seconds.

- Then turn your head back to the middle and face forward, stretching upward. Hold this position for a few seconds.

- Turn your head cautiously and slowly toward the left until you can feel it stretch. Hold that position for a few seconds.

- Then turn your head carefully and gradually all the way over to the right in one movement—do this while your head is facing the right side—and look over your right shoulder. While doing this, ensure that your back is straight and your shoulders are parallel with your feet.

- Finally, turn your head cautiously and slowly all the way over to the right in one movement—do this while your head is facing the right side—and look over your right shoulder.

- Start with two repetitions, gradually increasing per day, until you reach five repetitions.

Yoga as a Perfect Exercise to Manage Pain

If you want to have a more intensive physical activity that alleviates pain, the best option you have is to enroll in a yoga class. Yoga is a paradox of sorts: it is incredibly relaxing, and yet the workout that you receive is almost equivalent to one that you get while circuit training.

But the main reason why yoga works extremely well in relieving chronic pain is because it not only strengthens you physically, but mentally as well. The stretches and exercises give your physical body enough strength to combat the source of pain, while the meditative aspect helps your brain to accept and manage whatever discomfort you are feeling.

In the next chapter, you will see how the brain is as much responsible for handling pain as the body is.

Chapter Six
The Mind as the Best Painkiller

There are many cultures and languages in South East Asia, but most of them share this same proverb:

A man who accepts his wound will bear no pain at all;
A man who refuses will buckle under the slightest
scratch.

The mind is a powerful tool in combating pain. A strong mind with a strong will can withstand the most serious kinds of wounds and illnesses. You probably had a first-hand experience with this: that time when you had a terrible fever but felt better because of a big event (a first date; a party; graduation day); or that time when you complained of muscle aches but were able to accomplish the most impossible physical tasks.

This chapter will guide you to strengthening your mind in order to withstand and eventually be free from pain.

Belief in Healing Heals You

Believe it or not, one large factor why painkillers work so well is because of *your belief* that it would work. Extensive studies have been conducted by doctors and scientists that show the same results: the effect of painkillers is amplified or reduced by the person's attitude towards the drug.

In fact, several studies have already shown that even *without* real painkillers, a person's belief that he/she will feel well results in the materialization of that belief.

You've probably heard of the *placebo effect*, in which patients are given sugar pills instead of real pain relievers, and yet report an increase in wellbeing.

Well, recent studies have shown that the effect is not only psychological—it is also astoundingly physical.

Scientists from the University of Michigan have found that the patients who were given placebo and were led to believe that they received painkillers have an increase in endorphin levels. Endorphin is the body's natural internal painkiller. In contrast, patients who have received real painkillers have lower endorphin levels. The studies indicate that those who received true painkillers *are actually more prone to experiencing increased pain than those who received placebo.*

Your Mind can Control What You Feel

Still not a believer in the power of the mind? Then take the case of this study in 2005 at Stanford.

Laura Tibbits is a 33-year old who experienced chronic pain due to acquiring a severe fracture in her arm and shoulder blade several years ago. Doctors at Stanford asked Laura to be scanned by an MRI as she tries to control her pain levels.

The first thing she did is to try and make her pain worse. By reliving the injury, her pain levels shot up to 9 on a scale 10.

After which, she was instructed to think about reducing the pain that she feels. Laura imagined little people scooping out the pain that she was experiencing. Her pain levels decreased to 4 on a scale of 10, much lower than her levels when she started.

The study was replicated on several other subjects, and the results were the same. Subjects were able to decrease their pain levels by nearly two-thirds, all just by consciously willing it to reduce.

This study tells us that the mind is your most powerful tool against pain.

If you fear pain and consider it to be the worst thing in your life, you will probably intensify the discomfort you are already feeling. By accepting pain and treating it like something insignificant to be of any concern, you <u>will</u> significantly reduce the sensation.

Three Relaxation Techniques to Help Your Mind Combat Pain

You can easily reduce the pain that you are experiencing by doing relaxation exercises. These relaxation exercises shut down the signals responsible for pain, and increases endorphin production. Even if you do just one of these exercises once a day, it will help in gradually freeing you from pain.

Meditation

1. **Create your meditation space.** It need not be something so cliché as a room filled with scented candles and incense. You only need a room that has limited stimulus (quiet, not bright, not too colorful) and where you can be totally relaxed in. It can be your room, your couch, or your study. Some of my clients actually prefer to do their meditation in a bathtub, soaking in lukewarm water. You might want to try it yourself, as water is a great relaxant for your muscles.

2. **Ease yourself out of external stimuli.**
Remember how to properly prepare yourself
to sleep? You need to do a slightly similar thing
before meditation. Make sure your stomach
isn't full (but don't be hungry either), clean
yourself up a bit, and shut down all sources
of noise.

3. **Place yourself in the meditation space.** Make
sure to be in an upright yet comfortable position. Lying down will probably make you sleep
and will disrupt the meditation process, so it
is not advised.

4. **Relax your body.** Let all the tensions in your
muscle disappear. No part of your body should
feel like it's clenching something—if you feel
a muscle clench, let it loose. You should feel
your body getting lighter.

5. **Breathe gently.** *Gentle* is the keyword here. If
you breathe deeply and hard, your body will
not attain the state needed for meditation.

6. **Let go.** Loosen your mind's grip on your con-
cerns: no grocery lists, no deadlines, no past,
no future. Get into a state where there is only

now. You will know that you are in this state when you are fully relaxed and fully aware of your own self—as if your body is something foreign and new to you.

7. **Start turning your negativity to pain into something positive.** Once you are at a fully relaxed state, carefully feel the energy that is released by your body part that is experiencing pain. Accept this energy as something that is positive, as something that your body does to protect you. You can dwell on this as long as you need to.

8. **Release your aversions to healing.** You might be unconsciously holding yourself back to feeling better. If you hear thoughts such as "The pain will never go away," or "The pain will just keep coming back," now is the time to make these thoughts disappear. Do not fight these thoughts aggressively; be as gentle to it as you are to your pain.

9. **Experience your pain going away.** Note that I did not say *believe that your pain will go away*. In order for this meditation to work, you need

not only to believe in a future possibility, but also to will a present reality. Instead of telling yourself *I will be better*, say *I feel better already*. Stay on this state until you think your pain has reduced enough for this session.

10. **Ease in to external stimuli**. As you have started this meditation by easing in out of external stimuli, you also need your senses to gradually accept the things around them. Feel and smell the air around you. Listen to distant sounds. Imagine what your room looks like, and then slowly open your eyes. Maintain your meditative state for a few minutes with your senses fully open, before standing up and ending your session.

Guided Imagery

1. **Begin with your usual meditation preparation.** Designate a space, ease out of external stimuli, relax your body, breathe gently, and let go of your mind.

2. **Locate your pain.** Try to see yourself as an explorer of your body. You can use whatever

imagery you find to fit best to your personality. My client who was a sci-fi geek did this and told me she imagined herself as a captain of a spacecraft that was exploring her body. Imagine your internal organs: you can see your heart pumping out blood; your lungs inflating and deflating; your stomach churning. Now try and locate the source of pain. You might find that the most prevalent physical manifestation of pain might not be the real source—in that case, dig deep until you find it.

3. **Create an embodiment of pain.** Once you locate the source, try to picture a physical embodiment of pain in that source. Do not worry if the picture that pops into your mind is something that is so powerful and strong— you will always find ways to defeat it.

4. **Manifest objects, people, or entities that can help you defeat pain.** No matter how strong your pain looks, there is always something stronger than it. If you picture your pain as a raging fire, do your best to summon water to extinguish it. Don't worry if the image you conjure seems too silly. Enjoy the help being

given. My sci-fi geek of a client had a pool of acid as her image of pain; she told me that she imagined elemental dwarves made up of alkaline chemicals who helped her neutralize it.

5. **Clean up the remnants and start repairs.** In most cases, your image of pain would have destroyed a part of wherever it was seated. After you have extinguished pain, the next step would be to imagine repairing whatever it was that it damaged. Do not worry if you picture yourself doing a shoddy job at first; you can come back to this the next day and do a better job. Once you finish doing the repairs, you should be able to feel magnitudes better than when you started.

6. **Ease in to external stimuli.** Same as with meditation, but with an added flair: let your image of yourself out of your body before embracing the outside world.

Deep Breathing

1. **Assume a comfortable position.** Unlike meditation and guided imagery, you can do deep

breathing anywhere where you can be comfortable enough. You can either lie down or sit. When sitting down, make sure you have your back straight—don't slouch.

2. **Relax and close your eyes.** Loosen all stiff muscles and release all the tension that you have.

3. **Put one hand on top of your chest, and put the other on top of your belly.**

4. **Breathe normally.** Notice which part rises when you breathe: your chest or your belly? If it is your chest, you aren't breathing correctly. Try to breathe normally a few more times until you get the hang of breathing correctly to make your belly rise—this is called diaphragmatic breathing. When you are breathing like this, you are ingesting oxygen much more fully.

5. **Take slow, deep breaths.** Keep doing diaphragmatic breathing, but do it slowly. Fast deep breathing will only raise your heart rate, and will not help at all to ease your pain. Keep on breathing and you will eventually feel lighter—this is due to all the oxygen that you have allowed into your body. Continue doing it until you feel better.

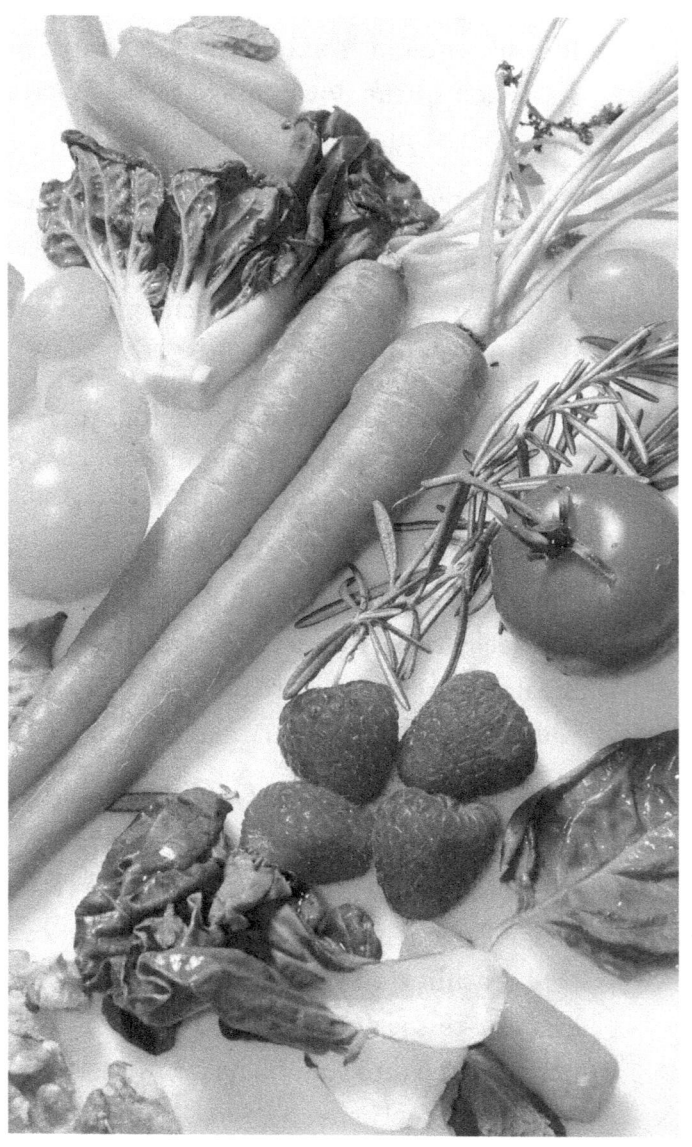

Chapter Seven

Nutrition as a Path to Feeling Well

Nutrition plays a vital role in alleviating your pain. The food, supplements, and vitamins that you take aid your body in recovering from injury, as well as in coping with pain.

To combat pain, you will need adequate amounts of nutrients as well as hormonal supplements. In this chapter, I will teach you the fundamentals of natural nutritional and hormonal support in order for you to alleviate pain easily.

Nutritional Supplements to Consider

Modern research shows that a handful of herbs as well as nutritional supplements are better options for pain control. It is revealed that, after comparing non-steroidal anti-inflammatory drugs (NSAIDs) to these nutraceuticals, several of them are as successful at pain relief while the others have few-to-no side effects. More often, these natural products cost less than most drugs.

Anti-inflammatory Herbs

WILLOW BARK

The original source of the salicylic acid used in making aspirin is the willow bark. A recent study that was performed on 228 people with lower back pain compared willow bark (240 mg salicin) with the anti-inflammatory drug Vioxx. (*Take note that Vioxx is removed out of the market because of its dangerous side effects for most people.*) The study showed that both were equally effective.

Moreover, willow bark is much safer as well as 40% less costly. The research emphasized that the daily dose of willow bark products should never be more than 240 mg of salicin.

Here are some of the things that willow bark can do for you:

- You can use willow barks as an antioxidant.

- Willow barks can slow down as well as prevent harmful chemical reactions inside your body.

- In addition, willow barks can slow the production of pain-causing chemicals. The good thing about this is that it doesn't give you adverse side-effects aside from minor allergies.

- If you are experiencing chest pains due to cardiovascular diseases or hypertension, willow bark can also act as your blood thinning agent aside from aspirin.

BOSWELLIA

The Boswellia (*Boswellia serrata*) plant is a very effective and essential anti-inflammatory pain reliever. It is a well-documented and well-researched herb medicine.

This herb does not have any side effects that can

cause ulcers and other stomach irritation compared to most NSAIDs.

The only known but rare side effects of this herb are mild nausea, skin rash, or loose stools. Medical studies even recommend that Boswellia is very safe even after several weeks of use.

If you plan to take Boswellia, make sure to follow the regular dose of around 150mg, three times a day. A dose of Boswellia contains around 37.5–65 percent of boswellic acids.

Here are some of the things that Boswellia can do for you:

- Boswellia can help reduce fever as well as help relax your muscle. The herb works on many of your tissues that include the digestive tract, the joints, the colon as well as the airways.

- Boswellia can also help reduce swelling for brain cancer cases.

GINGER

Ginger (*Zingiber officinale*) is more common as food, specifically as spice. However, you might not know that ginger has a very long history of use as an anti-nausea and anti-inflammatory medicine.

If you are to take ginger for your body pain, I recommend that you use one gram (about one-half teaspoon) of powdered ginger or up to 50 grams a day of lightly cooked or fresh root.

Here are some of the things that ginger can do for you:

- It decreases the production of three different varieties of chemicals that can cause inflammation.

- Ginger has also been proven to safely and effectively decrease the pain as well as disability associated with migraine headaches, muscle aches, and arthritis.

- Compared to over-the-counter prescribed NSAIDs, ginger emerges to have a protective advantage against stomach ulceration. It also doesn't have any major side-effects. The only contraindication of ginger would be blood thinning medications as well as drugs employed to cure gallstones.

DEVIL'S CLAW

The Devil's Claw (*Harpagophytum procumbens*) has an extensive history of medical uses and treatments for musculoskeletal problems. Recent studies have proven that the Devil's Claw is effective and safe for relief of mild to moderate pain.

What's more surprising is that the Devil's Claw has no adverse effects. These studies have documented that the people given Devil's claw experience the same relief from pain as those who were advised to use NSAIDs.

If you plan on taking the Devil's Claw, I recommend a daily dose of 30mg and 60mg of harpagoside. You should continue treatment in not less than four weeks.

BROMELAIN

This wonder herb remedy comes from the stem of the pineapple plant's mixture of digestive enzymes.

I recommend that you to take a daily dose of two or three 2400 mcg capsules. It is safe to be taken on an empty stomach for two to three times daily. Do take note that if you have an allergy to honeybee venom, or to pineapple or olive tree pollen, you may potentially get an allergic response to Bromelain. Always consult your doctor before administering this herb for alternative pain management.

Here are some of the things that bromelain can do for you:

- Bromelain can help lessen pain and inflammation due to surgery, trauma, arthritis, or sports injury.

- It also aids in healing the digestive lining of your stomach.

- Bromelain is a good treatment for reducing edema, inflammation and knee pains. It can improve physical function, stiffness, as well as your overall psychological well-being. On top of that, Bromelain is also known to speed-up and increase healing.

- It is a very safe and effective alternative in treating osteoarthritis of the knee and wrists.

- If you have difficulty breathing because of sinusitis, then Bromelain is a good cure for you as this decreases mucosal inflammation.

- Bromelain is critical in assisting the cancer drugs vincristine and 5-fluorouracil to work effectively.

- Bromelain can reinforce certain antibiotics. It can increase the action and power of said medicines.

CURCUMIN

The Curcumin (*Curcuma longa*) is the yellow-colored substance that comes from turmeric root. This herb has been used for thousands of years in Asian as well as East Indian cooking.

- I recommend that you use a maximum dose of 8000 mg of Curcumin daily for a period of 3 months for treatment of severe inflammation and chronic pain.

- Here are some of the things that it can do for you:

- You can use Curcumin as a very powerful antioxidant.

- It has anti-inflammatory effects for your acute injuries, and can reduce chronic inflammation.

- If you have wounds and pains in the lining of your colon, Curcumin can heal the wounds and relieve the pain by repairing the cells and tissues of that lining.

- It increases the effects of aspirin and other blood thinning drugs.

QUERCETIN

This is considered to be one of the most important plant medicines studied in recent years. Quercetin has a wide range of benefits for you: from treatment of chronic pain and inflammation to helping stop the spread of cancer to serving as an anti-viral prevention and cure.

This herb medicine is also widely distributed in nature so you can always get this in a lot of forms. You can obtain quercetin from green tea, apples, red onions, tomato, broccoli, red grapes, green leafy vegetables, and a number of berries such as raspberry, lingonberry, sweet rowan, cranberry and chokeberry.

Here are some of the things that quercetin can do for you:

- Quercetin can slow down histamine production as well as other inflammatory chemicals from your white blood cells.

- This herb can also significantly reduce acute inflammation as well as the swelling and pain of your arthritis.

- If you are experiencing fibromyalgia, you can best treat that with quercetin.

- Quercetin is definitely a good treatment for you if you have hypertension or if you are suffering from obesity.

- Quercetin is also proven to be effective against cancer.

Nutrients

VITAMIN D

If you are suffering from limb pain, chronic musculoskeletal pain, and lower back pain, it's likely that you lack significant levels of Vitamin D in your body.

You can supplement your Vitamin D deficiency through oral Vitamin D pills. Increasing Vitamin D levels in your body would provide you a lot of benefits, some of which are:

- Vitamin D can significantly reduce pains related to your musculoskeletal system safely.

- Vitamin D can give you safe and effective anti-inflammatory effects for acute and chronic pains all over your body.

- Vitamin D can give you a boost in resistance and cure to skin-related inflammations and pains.

I advise you to schedule an annual blood examination in order to gauge the Vitamin D levels in your body. This is to let you become aware if you need higher doses of Vitamin D or not.

While higher doses of Vitamin D may be safe for you, I don't recommend you to increase your consumption if you are also taking thiazide diuretics. Moreover, if you have a hypersensitive reaction to Vitamin D, it is best to skip the supplement. Hypersensitivity to Vitamin D would include manifestations of hypothyroidism, adrenal insufficiency, Crohn's disease as well as tuberculosis.

NIACINAMIDE

This nutritional supplement is a common type of vitamin B3. Oral Niacinamide supplements as well as Niacinamide therapy have become popular now in the field of rehabilitation medicine. More and more doctors are recommending the use of Niacinamide for pain management.

Niacinamide can provide you the following benefits:

- It is a highly effective treatment if you are suffering from osteoarthritis.

- It can also improve joint mobility.

- It can reduce any objective inflammation you are suffering from.

- It can also reduce the impact of your arthritis to your daily activities.

- It can reduce your use for pain medications.

- It can give you a calming effect, hence reducing your anxiety.

There are no known side effects of Niacinamine if you keep your daily doses well below 3000mg. But I suggest you have your liver check three months after you started Niacinamide treatment. That is to check that the supplement won't have any adverse reactions to your liver enzymes.

MSM (METHYLSULFONYLMETHANE)

The MSM has already been an established and popular nutritional supplement over the years.

You can use MSM for the following symptoms:

- Pain due to allergies

- Joint pains

- Interstitial cystitis

- Muscle pains

- Fatigue and exhaustion

The good thing about it is that MSM is it is really cheap and safe. I recommend a dose of 2600mg for a maximum of one month to relieve you of recurring bodily pains.

GLUCOSAMINE AND CHONDROITIN SULFATE

These two nutrients are considered to be the building blocks utilized for cartilage construction. The use of glucosamine and chondroitin sulfate as supplements has existed in the medical sciences for years.

Here are the following benefits you can get from making use of glucosamine and chondroitin as supplements:

- Slow down the breakage of joint cartilage caused by arthritis.

- Eliminates or reduces arthritis pains in your hands, knees, hips, lower back and jaw.

- Lessen the effects of rheumatic pains.

- Safe for treatment on osteoarthritis disability and pains.

I suggest you take a daily dose of glucosamine sulfate in between 1500 and 2000 mg. You should divide the dose probably two to three times daily. You can use chondroitin sulfate for 1,000 mg a day.

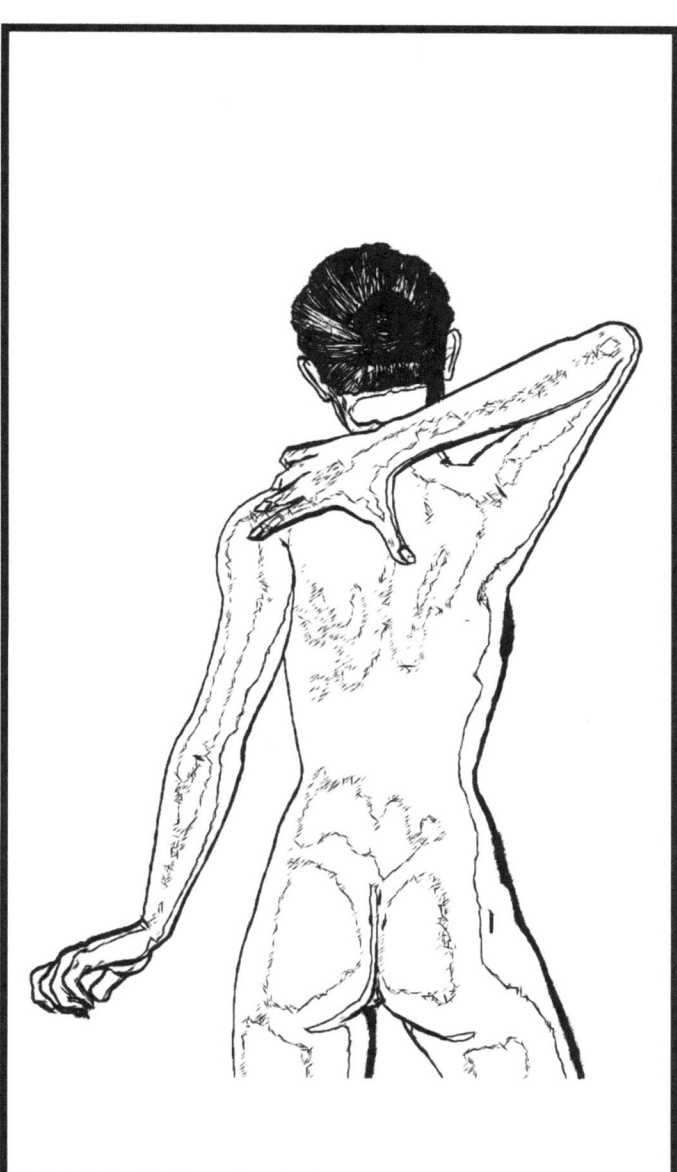

Fighting Inflammation

In this bonus chapter, we will explore the physical manifestation of pain: inflammation. Inflammation is when the affected part of your body—the part that is injured and the source of pain—displays redness and swelling. You often see this when you accidentally cut or bruise yourself.

Like pain, inflammation is not a bad thing in itself; it is a sign that your body is functioning well and appropriately to an injury. It is part of a healthy immune response. It is when inflammation is in excess that it becomes unhelpful, and indeed, harmful to your body.

This excess inflammation is abundant in our modern society; and what's worse, it is almost invisible. Low level chronic inflammation is not as noticeable as the inflammation you get from a wound or bruise; in fact, you would only notice the after effects: heart disease, diabetes, osteoporosis, and mood disorders, among others.

The good thing is that you can fight the excess inflammation through simple diet and lifestyle adjustments. If you combine these tricks with the five simple steps that I have outlined in the past chapters, you are on your way to living the rest of your life healthy and truly pain-free.

Managing Inflammation through Proper Diet

Chronic inflammation is usually triggered by having an unbalanced diet. Most people eat too many food items that induce the production of inflammatory chemicals in their body. A diet that is comprised of too many processed foods, most of which lack antioxidants and also make the immune system less efficient.

Here are some of the items that you should be taking in moderation:

- Food with trans fats, saturated fats, and hydrogenated oils

- Food that have refined carbohydrates

- Conventionally produced animal products are especially high in arachidonic acid, which triggers the inflammatory response

- Solanine found in plants from the nightshade family (potato, tomatoes, eggplants)

- You don't need to completely avoid the food items listed above; that is almost impossible in modern society. What you need to do is balance it with items that quell inflammation:

- Food that contain healthy fats, such as omega-3 fatty acids which can be found in wild-caught salmon, herring, and mackerel

- Antioxidant-rich items, such as onion, blueberries, sweet potatoes, spinach, and pineapples

- Spices that boost your immune system like garlic, turmeric, cinnamon, and clove

Managing Inflammation with Cold

If your pain due to chronic inflammation is hindering you from following the five steps outlined in the previous chapters, you might have to address the inflammation first. If you cannot meditate, sleep, or exercise because of your arthritis, cooling the inflamed part should be the first thing you do.

Simply grab an ice pack and apply it on the affected area. Cold water isn't enough; the cooling effect is achieved through conduction, and is more effective as the temperature difference between the coolant and the inflamed part increases.

One thing you should understand about cooling an inflammation is that you are not aiming to transfer the cold to the tissues, but to make heat from the tissues come out.

Apply the ice pack for around 15 to 30 minutes. The inflamed area should be a bit better now, enough for you to continue with exercising or focus on meditation.

Conclusion
The Responsibilities of Maintaining a Pain-Free Life

Most of you who are reading this book will probably find your pain reduced significantly after just a week or even just a few days of doing the five simple steps. You will probably ask yourself why you've been dosing on painkillers for how many years now, if the solution is really that simple.

There is actually one more trick to make the five simple steps work at its maximum. With this trick, you will not only reduce pain, but you will really, truly, break free from it.

Do you want to know what the trick is?

Consistency.

It is such a simple trick. In order for you to truly break free from pain, you need to do the five simple steps consistently, without fail.

The five simple steps are not instant cures, and they are not a one-off deal. When you do the five steps only whenever you feel pain, you've missed out on the chance to fully realize its potential.

The reason why those simple steps are so effective in reducing your pain is because it helps your body at what it naturally does. The reason why it is so effective is because that is really how you should have been living your life from the start: drinking enough water, getting plenty of sleep, exercising, being in touch with your inner self, and eating healthily.

This book is only the beginning. Be consistent with the five simple steps, and you will not only break free from pain, you will also enter into a whole new energized life.

A note about links. We've included a lot of links to external information in this book. Realize that links do go out of date. If a link is out of date, please let us know by emailing us and we will update it in the next version.

Reviews are very important for the success of a book. If you enjoyed *Pain Relief: The Drug-Free Way to Feel Better Fast*, please leave a review (http://amzn.to/2fBrIk9). Even a few words helps.

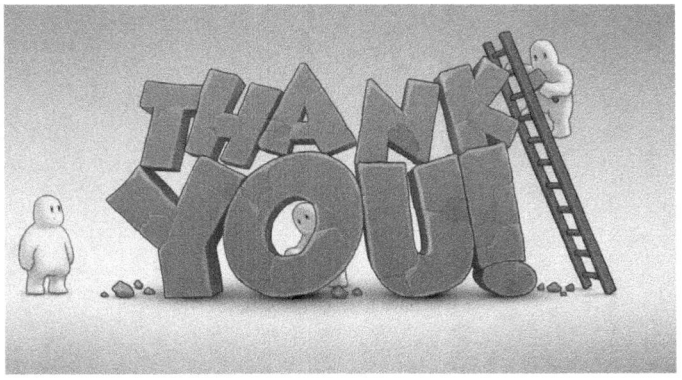